I0696255

Table of Contents

Chapter 1: Understanding Hashimoto's Thyroiditis

Introduction:

Hashimoto's Thyroiditis is an autoimmune condition that affects the thyroid gland, causing inflammation and interfering with its ability to produce essential hormones. In this chapter, we will delve into the intricacies of Hashimoto's Thyroiditis, exploring its causes, symptoms, and the impact of diet on managing the condition effectively.

What is Hashimoto's Thyroiditis?

Hashimoto's Thyroiditis is named after Dr. Hakaru Hashimoto, a Japanese physician who first described the condition in 1912. It is the most common cause of hypothyroidism, characterized by the immune system mistakenly attacking the thyroid gland. This autoimmune response leads to chronic inflammation and gradual destruction of thyroid tissue, impairing its function.

Within the thyroid gland, follicular cells produce two vital hormones: triiodothyronine (T3) and thyroxine (T4). These hormones regulate metabolism, energy levels, growth, and development. In Hashimoto's Thyroiditis, the immune system produces antibodies that target and damage these cells, disrupting the production and release of T3 and T4.

Causes and Risk Factors

The exact cause of Hashimoto's Thyroiditis remains unclear, but a combination of genetic and environmental factors is believed to play a role. Genetic predisposition, family history, and gender (women are more prone to the condition) contribute to the risk factors. Furthermore, certain environmental triggers, such as viral infections, stress, and hormonal imbalances, can activate or exacerbate the autoimmune response.

Symptoms and Diagnosis

Hashimoto's Thyroiditis often develops gradually, making it challenging to recognize in its early stages. Symptoms can vary widely from person to person and may be subtle at first. Common symptoms include fatigue, weight gain, sensitivity to cold, dry skin, constipation, hair loss, and muscle weakness.

To diagnose Hashimoto's Thyroiditis, healthcare professionals typically conduct a thorough medical history assessment, physical examination, and blood tests to measure thyroid hormone levels and the presence of specific antibodies, such as anti-thyroid peroxidase (anti-TPO) and anti-thyroglobulin (anti-Tg) antibodies.

The Impact of Diet on Hashimoto's Thyroiditis

Diet plays a crucial role in managing Hashimoto's Thyroiditis and optimizing thyroid function. While diet alone cannot cure the condition, it can significantly impact symptoms, inflammation levels, and overall well-being. Certain dietary factors can either support or hinder thyroid function.

Several nutrients are particularly important for thyroid health, including iodine, selenium, zinc, iron, and vitamins A, D, and B12. Iodine is essential for the production of thyroid hormones, but excessive intake can trigger autoimmune thyroiditis in susceptible individuals. Selenium, on the other hand, has been shown to reduce thyroid inflammation and improve thyroid antibody levels.

In addition to specific nutrients, the overall quality of the diet is crucial. A diet rich in whole, unprocessed foods, ample fruits and vegetables, lean proteins, and healthy fats can provide essential nutrients and support the immune system. On the other hand, a diet high in processed foods, refined sugars, unhealthy fats, and food allergens can promote inflammation and worsen symptoms.

Understanding the connection between diet and Hashimoto's Thyroiditis sets the foundation for the subsequent chapters of this book, which will explore dietary strategies, meal plans, and lifestyle modifications to support thyroid health and manage the condition effectively.

By gaining a comprehensive understanding of Hashimoto's Thyroiditis, its causes, symptoms, and the influence of diet, you are now equipped with the knowledge to embark on a transformative journey towards improved well-being and thyroid management. In the following chapters, we will dive deeper into the foundations of the Hashimoto Diet, creating a healing environment, and implementing specific dietary guidelines and meal plans to support your thyroid health.

Chapter 2: Foundations of the Hashimoto Diet

Introduction:

In this chapter, we will explore the fundamental principles of the Hashimoto Diet and understand how nutrition plays a pivotal role in managing Hashimoto's Thyroiditis. By focusing on key nutrients, potential triggers, and allergens, you will gain insights into building a strong foundation for your dietary approach and optimizing your thyroid health.

Section 2.1: The Role of Nutrition in Managing Hashimoto's Thyroiditis

Nutrition is a powerful tool for managing Hashimoto's Thyroiditis as it can influence thyroid function, reduce inflammation, and support the immune system. A well-balanced diet can provide essential nutrients that are crucial for thyroid health and overall well-being.

Understanding the impact of nutrition on Hashimoto's Thyroiditis empowers you to make informed choices about the foods you consume and how they can either support or hinder your thyroid function. By adopting a proactive approach to nutrition, you can take control of your health and improve your quality of life.

Section 2.2: Key Nutrients for Thyroid Health

Several nutrients play a vital role in supporting optimal thyroid function. These include iodine, selenium, zinc, iron, and vitamins A, D, and B12. Iodine is essential for the production of thyroid hormones, but it's crucial to strike a balance as excessive intake can trigger autoimmune thyroiditis in susceptible individuals.

Selenium is a powerful antioxidant that helps reduce inflammation and support the immune system. It has been shown to improve thyroid antibody levels and decrease thyroid peroxidase (TPO) antibodies in people with Hashimoto's Thyroiditis. Including selenium-rich foods like

Brazil nuts, seafood, and organ meats in your diet can be beneficial.

Zinc and iron are necessary for the synthesis and activation of thyroid hormones. Deficiencies in these minerals can impair thyroid function and exacerbate symptoms of Hashimoto's Thyroiditis. Foods such as lean meats, seafood, legumes, nuts, and seeds are excellent sources of zinc and iron.

Vitamins A, D, and B12 also play essential roles in thyroid health. Vitamin A supports the production and conversion of thyroid hormones, while vitamin D regulates immune function and may help modulate autoimmune responses. Vitamin

B12 is involved in energy production and supports nerve health.

Section 2.3: Potential Triggers and Allergens

Certain foods and substances can potentially trigger or worsen symptoms in individuals with Hashimoto's Thyroiditis. Identifying and eliminating these triggers can be a key strategy for managing the condition effectively.

Gluten, a protein found in wheat and related grains, has been implicated in autoimmune thyroid disorders. Many people with Hashimoto's Thyroiditis find that removing gluten from their diet improves their symptoms. Similarly, dairy products, soy, and processed foods containing artificial additives may also contribute to inflammation and exacerbate thyroid-related symptoms.

Food allergies and sensitivities can also have a significant impact on Hashimoto's Thyroiditis. Common allergens such as eggs, nuts, shellfish, and nightshade vegetables (e.g., tomatoes, potatoes, peppers) may trigger immune responses and worsen symptoms. Identifying and avoiding these allergens can be crucial for symptom management.

Elimination diets and reintroduction protocols can help identify specific triggers and allergens. By systematically removing potential culprits from your diet and reintroducing them one by one, you can determine which foods contribute to your symptoms and make informed decisions about your dietary choices.

Understanding the role of key nutrients, potential triggers, and allergens empowers you to make proactive choices when it comes to your diet. By incorporating foods rich in essential nutrients and avoiding potential triggers, you can create a solid foundation for your Hashimoto Diet journey.

As we move forward in the subsequent chapters, we will delve deeper into the practical aspects of the Hashimoto Diet, exploring food preparation techniques, meal planning, and personalized diet maintenance. By implementing these strategies, you will be well on your way to optimizing your thyroid health and reclaiming your vitality.

Chapter 3: Creating a Healing Environment

Introduction:

In Chapter 3, we will explore the importance of creating a healing environment for managing Hashimoto's Thyroiditis. Beyond dietary considerations, lifestyle factors, stress reduction techniques, sleep, exercise, and other lifestyle modifications all play crucial roles in supporting thyroid health and overall well-being. By adopting a holistic approach, you can enhance the effectiveness of your Hashimoto Diet and improve your quality of life.

Section 3.1: Lifestyle Factors for Managing Hashimoto's Thyroiditis

Lifestyle factors have a significant impact on Hashimoto's Thyroiditis and can either support or undermine your efforts to manage the condition. By addressing certain aspects of your daily routine, you can create a healing environment that promotes optimal thyroid function.

One critical aspect is managing stress. Chronic stress can trigger and exacerbate autoimmune responses, leading to increased inflammation and worsening of symptoms. Implementing stress reduction techniques such as mindfulness meditation, deep breathing exercises, yoga, and engaging in hobbies or activities that bring you joy can help alleviate stress and support your overall well-being.

Sleep plays a vital role in hormone regulation and immune function. Getting sufficient, restful sleep is essential for managing Hashimoto's Thyroiditis. Establishing a regular sleep schedule, creating a calming sleep environment, and practicing good sleep hygiene can contribute to improved thyroid health and overall vitality.

Maintaining a healthy weight is also important for managing Hashimoto's Thyroiditis. Excess weight can put additional strain on the thyroid gland and exacerbate symptoms. Adopting a balanced, nutrient-dense diet, engaging in regular physical activity, and seeking support from healthcare professionals or registered dietitians can help you achieve and maintain a healthy weight.

Section 3.2: Reducing Stress and Managing Cortisol Levels

Stress reduction is a key component of managing Hashimoto's Thyroiditis. Chronic stress can dysregulate cortisol levels, the primary stress hormone, which can have adverse effects on thyroid function and immune responses.

Implementing stress management techniques can help regulate cortisol levels and support overall well-being. Mindfulness meditation, for example, has been shown to reduce stress, promote relaxation, and support a healthy stress response. By incorporating mindfulness practices into your daily routine, you can cultivate a sense of calm and balance in your life.

Regular exercise is another effective way to manage stress and support thyroid health. Engaging in physical activity releases endorphins, which are natural mood-boosting chemicals. Exercise also improves blood circulation, promotes detoxification, and supports overall vitality. Finding activities you enjoy, such as walking, cycling, swimming, or dancing, can make exercise an enjoyable and sustainable part of your lifestyle.

Section 3.3: Sleep, Exercise, and Other Lifestyle Considerations

In addition to stress reduction techniques, focusing on quality sleep and regular exercise can have profound effects on managing Hashimoto's Thyroiditis.

Creating a sleep-friendly environment involves optimizing your bedroom for relaxation and rest. This includes keeping the room cool, dark, and quiet, and avoiding electronic devices before bedtime. Establishing a consistent sleep routine and practicing relaxation techniques, such as gentle stretching or reading a book, can help signal your body to wind down and prepare for sleep.

When it comes to exercise, finding a balance is key. Moderate-intensity exercises, such as brisk walking, cycling, or yoga, can provide numerous benefits for thyroid health without overtaxing the body. Listen to your body's cues and adjust the intensity and duration of your workouts accordingly.

Beyond stress reduction, sleep, and exercise, other lifestyle considerations can support your healing journey. These include minimizing exposure to environmental toxins, such as chemicals in cleaning products and personal care items, as they can disrupt hormone function. Opting for natural, organic alternatives and creating a toxin-free home environment can promote better thyroid health.

Additionally, seeking support from healthcare professionals, joining support groups, or connecting with others who have Hashimoto's Thyroiditis can provide a sense of community and emotional support. Sharing experiences, tips, and strategies can be invaluable in navigating the challenges of managing the condition.

By addressing lifestyle factors, reducing stress, optimizing sleep, incorporating regular exercise, and making conscious choices to create a healing environment, you are empowering yourself to manage Hashimoto's Thyroiditis more effectively. These lifestyle modifications, in conjunction with the dietary strategies discussed in previous chapters, will set the stage for improved thyroid health and overall well-being.

As we progress to the following chapters, we will explore the practical aspects of the Hashimoto Diet, including guidelines for choosing the right foods, meal planning tips, and delicious recipes that promote optimal thyroid function. By incorporating these strategies into your daily life, you will be well on your way to thriving with Hashimoto's Thyroiditis.

Chapter 4: The Hashimoto Diet: Guidelines and Principles

Introduction:

In Chapter 4, we will delve into the guidelines and principles of the Hashimoto Diet, which will serve as a blueprint for optimizing your nutrition and managing Hashimoto's Thyroiditis. We will explore the importance of choosing the right foods, maintaining macronutrient balance, portion control, and implementing effective food preparation and cooking techniques. By following these guidelines, you will create a nourishing and supportive dietary approach for your thyroid health.

Section 4.1: Choosing the Right Foods

Choosing the right foods is fundamental to the Hashimoto Diet. It involves selecting nutrient-dense, whole foods that support thyroid function, reduce inflammation, and provide the body with essential vitamins, minerals, and antioxidants.

Aim to include a wide variety of fruits and vegetables in your diet, as they are rich in antioxidants that help combat inflammation and oxidative stress. Dark leafy greens, such as spinach and kale, are particularly beneficial due to their high nutrient content.

Incorporating lean proteins, such as poultry, fish, eggs, and legumes, provides essential amino acids for thyroid hormone synthesis and overall cellular health. Healthy fats, including avocados, nuts, seeds, and olive oil, are important for hormone production and absorption of fat-soluble vitamins.

When it comes to carbohydrates, focus on complex carbohydrates like whole grains, quinoa, and sweet potatoes. These provide sustained energy and fiber, which promotes gut health and supports proper digestion.

Section 4.2: Macronutrient Balance and Portion Control

Maintaining a proper macronutrient balance is essential for managing Hashimoto's Thyroiditis. Balancing carbohydrates, proteins, and fats helps regulate blood sugar levels, supports hormone production, and optimizes energy levels.

Consider incorporating the plate method as a guideline for portion control. Fill half your plate with non-starchy vegetables, one-quarter with lean protein, and one-quarter with complex carbohydrates. This ensures a balanced meal that provides essential nutrients and supports stable blood sugar levels.

Pay attention to portion sizes and listen to your body's hunger and fullness cues. Overeating can lead to weight gain and strain on the thyroid, while undereating can deprive the body of essential nutrients. Aim for a balanced and mindful approach to eating, allowing yourself to enjoy meals while being mindful of portion sizes.

Section 4.3: Food Preparation and Cooking Techniques

Food preparation and cooking techniques can greatly impact the nutritional quality of your meals. Opting for healthier cooking methods can help preserve nutrients and promote optimal thyroid health.

Consider using cooking methods such as steaming, sautéing, grilling, or baking instead of deep frying. These methods require less added fat and retain the natural flavors and nutrients of the ingredients.

When it comes to food preparation, try to consume a mix of raw and cooked foods. While cooking can enhance the flavors and textures of certain ingredients, raw foods, such as salads and smoothies, provide a fresh and vibrant source of enzymes, vitamins, and minerals.

Experiment with herbs, spices, and seasonings to add flavor to your meals without relying on excessive salt or unhealthy condiments. Fresh herbs like basil, cilantro, and parsley, as well as spices like turmeric, cumin, and ginger, not only add delicious flavors but also offer anti-inflammatory and antioxidant properties.

Section 4.4: Meal Planning and Grocery Shopping Tips

Meal planning and smart grocery shopping are crucial components of the Hashimoto Diet. By being prepared and organized, you can make healthier choices and ensure that your kitchen is stocked with nutritious ingredients.

When meal planning, consider incorporating a variety of colors and textures into your meals to ensure a diverse range of nutrients. Make a list of the meals you plan to prepare for the week, including breakfast, lunch, dinner, and snacks. This will help you stay organized, save time, and make healthier choices.

When grocery shopping, focus on the perimeter of the store, where fresh produce, lean proteins, and whole grains are typically located. Avoid the middle aisles that often contain processed and packaged foods. Opt for organic and locally sourced options whenever possible to reduce exposure to pesticides and support sustainable farming practices.

Consider batch cooking and meal prepping on weekends or whenever you have some free time. This allows you to prepare larger quantities of meals and portion them out for the week. It can save time and ensure that you always have healthy, homemade options readily available.

By following these guidelines for choosing the right foods, maintaining macronutrient balance, practicing portion control, and adopting effective food preparation and cooking techniques, you will create a solid foundation for your Hashimoto Diet journey. In the next chapter, we will explore a comprehensive meal plan that incorporates these principles and provides delicious and nutritious recipes to support your thyroid health and overall well-being.

Chapter 5: The Hashimoto Diet Meal Plan

Introduction:

In Chapter 5, we will embark on a comprehensive journey into the Hashimoto Diet Meal Plan. This meal plan is designed to provide you with practical guidance, delicious recipes, and a structured approach to optimizing your nutrition and managing Hashimoto's Thyroiditis. We will explore three phases: the Elimination Phase, the Reintroduction Phase, and the Personalized Diet Maintenance Phase. By following this meal plan, you will be able to tailor your diet to suit your individual needs and support your thyroid health effectively.

Section 5.1: Phase 1: Elimination Phase

The Elimination Phase is the initial stage of the Hashimoto Diet Meal Plan. It involves temporarily eliminating potential trigger foods and common allergens to reduce inflammation, identify food sensitivities, and establish a foundation for personalized dietary modifications.

During this phase, you will eliminate gluten-containing grains (wheat, barley, rye), dairy products, soy, processed foods, refined sugars, and unhealthy fats. Instead, focus on whole, unprocessed foods such as lean proteins, fruits, vegetables, nuts, seeds, and gluten-free grains like quinoa and brown rice.

Emphasize nutrient-dense foods that support thyroid health, such as seaweed, Brazil nuts (for selenium), and leafy greens (for vitamins and minerals). Experiment with various herbs and spices to enhance flavors without relying on common allergens or trigger foods.

The Elimination Phase typically lasts for a few weeks, allowing your body to heal and reset. During this time, pay close attention to how you feel, noting any improvements in symptoms and energy levels. This will provide valuable insights for the next phase.

Section 5.2: Phase 2: Reintroduction Phase

After the Elimination Phase, you will enter the Reintroduction Phase, where you systematically reintroduce eliminated foods one by one to identify any potential triggers or food sensitivities. This phase helps you personalize your diet based on your individual tolerance and needs.

Start by reintroducing one eliminated food at a time, in small portions, and monitor your body's response over the next few days. Note any changes in symptoms, digestion, energy levels, or overall well-being. This step-by-step process allows you to identify specific foods that may trigger negative reactions.

For example, you might reintroduce gluten-containing grains first and observe how your body reacts. If you experience adverse effects, it may indicate gluten sensitivity or intolerance. If no symptoms arise, you can proceed to reintroduce dairy, soy, or other eliminated foods in a similar manner.

Keep in mind that food sensitivities can vary among individuals, so it's important to pay attention to your body's unique responses. Consult with a healthcare professional or registered dietitian for guidance during this phase to ensure you are reintroducing foods safely and effectively.

Section 5.3: Phase 3: Personalized Diet Maintenance

Once you have completed the Reintroduction Phase and identified your trigger foods and sensitivities, you can enter the Personalized Diet Maintenance Phase. This phase allows you to tailor your diet based on your individual needs, preferences, and identified food sensitivities.

Based on the results of your reintroduction phase, you can make informed decisions about which foods to include, limit, or avoid. Customize your diet to include nutrient-dense foods that support your thyroid health while minimizing or eliminating foods that trigger negative reactions.

Meal planning and preparation become key in the Personalized Diet Maintenance Phase. Create a balanced meal plan that incorporates a variety of whole foods, lean proteins, healthy fats, and gluten-free grains. Consider using the plate method discussed in Chapter 4 to ensure macronutrient balance and portion control.

Explore new recipes and experiment with different cooking techniques to make your meals exciting and enjoyable. Engage in batch cooking and meal prepping to save time and ensure that you always have nourishing options readily available.

Section 5.4: Sample Meal Plans and Recipes

To further assist you in implementing the Hashimoto Diet Meal Plan, this section provides sample meal plans and a selection of delicious recipes. These meal plans offer a framework for creating balanced and satisfying meals that promote optimal thyroid function and overall well-being.

Each meal plan includes breakfast, lunch, dinner, and snack options. They incorporate a variety of foods, flavors, and cooking techniques to keep your meals interesting and enjoyable. The recipes feature nutrient-dense ingredients, herbs, and spices that support thyroid health and add depth to your culinary experience.

Feel free to adapt the meal plans and recipes based on your individual preferences, dietary restrictions, and identified food sensitivities. This is your opportunity to personalize your diet and make it a sustainable and enjoyable lifestyle choice.

By following the Hashimoto Diet Meal Plan, you will not only nourish your body with thyroid-supportive foods but also embark on a culinary adventure filled with flavors, textures, and satisfaction. With dedication and a willingness to explore new recipes and ingredients, you can optimize your nutrition and thrive with Hashimoto's Thyroiditis.

As we proceed to the following chapters, we will further expand on managing food sensitivities and allergies, exploring superfoods for thyroid health, and providing guidance on dining out and social situations. By incorporating these additional strategies into your Hashimoto Diet journey, you will be equipped with a comprehensive toolkit for managing your condition effectively.

Chapter 7: Superfoods for Thyroid Health

Introduction:

In Chapter 7, we will explore the concept of superfoods and their role in supporting thyroid health. Superfoods are nutrient-dense foods that offer exceptional health benefits due to their high content of vitamins, minerals, antioxidants, and other bioactive compounds. By incorporating these superfoods into your Hashimoto Diet, you can provide your thyroid with the essential nutrients it needs to function optimally. Get ready to discover a world of vibrant, flavorful, and nourishing foods that will elevate your thyroid health to new heights.

Section 7.1: Foods Rich in Essential Nutrients for the Thyroid

Certain foods are rich in the essential nutrients that support thyroid function. Including these nutrient-dense foods in your diet can help optimize thyroid health and promote overall well-being.

Iodine is a key nutrient for thyroid health as it is required for the synthesis of thyroid hormones. Sea vegetables, such as nori, kelp, and dulse, are excellent sources of iodine. Including these sea vegetables in your meals can ensure an adequate intake of this crucial mineral.

Selenium is another vital nutrient for the thyroid, as it helps protect the gland from oxidative damage and supports the conversion of T4 to T3, the active form of thyroid hormone. Brazil nuts are an exceptionally rich source of selenium. Just a few nuts a day can provide your body with the recommended daily intake of this important mineral.

Zinc is essential for the production and regulation of thyroid hormones. Foods such as oysters, beef, pumpkin seeds, and chickpeas are excellent sources of zinc. Including these foods in your diet can help maintain optimal zinc levels and support thyroid function.

Iron is necessary for the production of thyroid hormones and the transportation of oxygen throughout the body. Incorporate iron-rich foods such as lean meats, shellfish, legumes, and dark leafy greens into your meals to ensure adequate iron intake.

Vitamins A, D, and B12 also play critical roles in thyroid health. Foods such as carrots, sweet potatoes, spinach, fatty fish (e.g., salmon, mackerel), eggs, and grass-fed beef are rich sources of these vitamins. Including these foods in your diet can provide the necessary nutrients for optimal thyroid function.

Section 7.2: Antioxidant-Rich Foods and Their Benefits

Antioxidants play a crucial role in protecting the thyroid gland from oxidative stress and reducing inflammation. Including antioxidant-rich foods in your diet can help support thyroid health and overall well-being.

Berries, such as blueberries, strawberries, and raspberries, are packed with antioxidants that combat free radicals and reduce inflammation. They are also rich in vitamins, minerals, and fiber, making them an excellent choice for promoting thyroid health.

Cruciferous vegetables, including broccoli, cauliflower, Brussels sprouts, and cabbage, contain compounds called glucosinolates. These compounds have been shown to support the liver's detoxification processes, which can indirectly benefit the thyroid. Cooking these vegetables can help deactivate enzymes that interfere with thyroid function.

Turmeric, a bright yellow spice, contains a powerful antioxidant compound called curcumin. Curcumin has been found to possess anti-inflammatory properties and may help modulate the immune response. Incorporating turmeric into your cooking or enjoying it as a tea can offer potential benefits for thyroid health.

Green tea is another antioxidant-rich beverage that may have positive effects on the thyroid. It contains polyphenols, such as epigallocatechin gallate (EGCG), which has been shown to have anti-inflammatory and antioxidant properties. Drinking green tea in moderation can be a refreshing way to support your thyroid health.

Section 7.3: Herbs and Supplements for Supporting Thyroid Function

In addition to superfoods, certain herbs and supplements can provide additional support for thyroid function. While it is important to consult with a healthcare professional or registered dietitian before starting any new supplements, incorporating these options into your diet may be beneficial.

Ashwagandha is an adaptogenic herb known for its stress-reducing properties. It may help support adrenal function and modulate cortisol levels, which can indirectly benefit thyroid health. Consider incorporating ashwagandha into your diet through herbal tea, capsules, or as an ingredient in recipes.

Probiotics are beneficial bacteria that promote gut health and support the immune system. Maintaining a healthy gut microbiome is crucial for overall well-being, including thyroid health.

Include probiotic-rich foods like yogurt, kefir, sauerkraut, and kimchi in your diet or consider taking a high-quality probiotic supplement.

Omega-3 fatty acids, found in fatty fish like salmon, mackerel, and sardines, have anti-inflammatory properties and may support thyroid health. If you are not consuming enough omega-3-rich foods, you can consider adding a high-quality fish oil supplement to your routine. However, consult with a healthcare professional before starting any new supplements.

It's important to note that while these herbs and supplements may offer potential benefits, they should not replace a nutrient-rich diet or medical treatment. Always consult with a healthcare professional before adding any new herbs or supplements to your routine, as they can interact with medications or have contraindications for certain conditions.

By incorporating superfoods rich in essential nutrients, antioxidant-rich foods, and herbs and supplements that support thyroid function, you can optimize your Hashimoto Diet and nourish your thyroid gland. These foods and supplements not only offer potential benefits for thyroid health but also add exciting flavors and textures to your meals, making your culinary experience enjoyable and satisfying.

As we proceed to the following chapters, we will explore strategies for managing dining out and social situations, tracking and monitoring your progress, and incorporating complementary therapies and alternative medicine into your Hashimoto Diet journey. By incorporating these additional strategies, you will have a comprehensive toolkit to support your thyroid health and overall well-being.

Hashimoto's Thyroiditis

Also called Hashimoto's disease, Hashimoto's thyroiditis is an autoimmune disease, a disorder in which the immune system turns against the body's own tissues. In people with Hashimoto's, the immune system attacks the thyroid. This can lead to hypothyroidism, a condition in which the thyroid does not make enough hormones for the body's needs.

Located in the front of your neck, the thyroid gland makes hormones that control metabolism. This includes your heart rate and how quickly your body uses calories from the foods you eat.

Causes of Hashimoto's Thyroiditis

The exact cause of Hashimoto's is not known, but many factors are believed to play a role. They include:

Genes. People who get Hashimoto's often have family members who have thyroid disease or other autoimmune diseases. This suggests a genetic component to the disease.

Hormones. Hashimoto's affects about seven times as many women as men, suggesting that sex hormones may play a role. Furthermore, some women have thyroid problems during the first year after having a baby. Although the problem usually goes away, as many as 20% of these women develop Hashimoto's years later.

Excessive iodine. Research suggests certain drugs and too much iodine, a trace element required by your body to make thyroid hormones, may trigger thyroid disease in susceptible people.

Radiation exposure. Increased cases of thyroid disease have been reported in people exposed to radiation, including the atomic bombs in Japan, the Chernobyl nuclear accident, and radiation treatment for a form of blood cancer called Hodgkin's disease.

Symptoms of Hashimoto's Thyroiditis

Hashimoto's symptoms may be mild at first or take years to develop. The first sign of the disease is often an enlarged thyroid, called a goiter. The goiter may cause the front of your neck to look swollen. A large goiter may make swallowing difficult. Other symptoms of an underactive thyroid due to Hashimoto's may include:

- Weight gain

- Fatigue

- Paleness or puffiness of the face

- Joint and muscle pain

- Constipation

- Inability to get warm

- Difficulty getting pregnant

- Hair loss or thinning, brittle hair

- Irregular or heavy menstrual periods

- Depression

- Slowed heart rate

Because the symptoms of Hashimoto's thyroid may be similar to those for other medical conditions, it is important to see your doctor for a diagnosis.

Treatments for Hashimoto's Thyroiditis

There is no cure for Hashimoto's, but replacing hormones with medication can regulate hormone levels and restore your normal metabolism.

The pills are available in several different strengths. The exact dose your doctor prescribes will depend on a number of factors, including:

- Age

- Weight

- Severity of hypothyroidism

- Other health problems

- Other medicines that may interact with synthetic thyroid hormones

Once you start treatment, your doctor will order a lab test called a thyroid-stimulating hormone (TSH) test to monitor thyroid function and help ensure you are getting the right dose. Because thyroid hormones act very slowly in the body, it may take a few months for symptoms to go away and your goiter to shrink. However, large goiters that do not improve may make it necessary to remove the thyroid gland.

Hashimoto Diet: Overview, Foods, Supplements, and Tips

Hashimoto's (or Hashimoto) thyroiditis — also called Hashimoto's disease — is one of the most common thyroid disorders in the United States and other developed countries.

Even when treated with medication, its symptoms may significantly affect quality of life.

Research shows that diet and lifestyle modifications may drastically improve symptoms, in addition to standard medication. Every person with Hashimoto's disease responds differently to treatment, which is why an individualized approach for this condition is so important.

This article explains the diet and lifestyle modifications most likely to benefit those with Hashimoto's disease.

Hashimoto's disease overview

Hashimoto's thyroiditis is an autoimmune disease that gradually destroys thyroid tissue via lymphocytes, which are white blood cells that are part of your immune system.

The thyroid is a butterfly-shaped endocrine gland that sits at the base of your neck. It secretes hormones that affect nearly every organ system, including your heart, lungs, skeleton, and digestive and central nervous systems. It also controls metabolism and growth.

The main hormones secreted by the thyroid are thyroxine (T4) and triiodothyronine (T3).

Eventually, damage to this gland leads to insufficient thyroid hormone production.

SUMMARY

Hashimoto's disease is an autoimmune condition that affects your thyroid, eventually causing inadequate hormone production.

How diet and lifestyle affect Hashimoto's

Diet and lifestyle play vital roles in managing Hashimoto's, as numerous individuals find that their symptoms persist even with medication. Plus, many people who exhibit symptoms aren't given medication unless they have altered hormone levels.

What's more, research suggests that inflammation may be a driving factor behind the wide range of Hashimoto's symptoms. Inflammation is often tied to diet.

Diet and lifestyle modifications are likewise key to reducing your risk of other ailments, as people with Hashimoto's disease have a higher risk of developing autoimmune conditions, high cholesterol, obesity, and diabetes.

Research shows that cutting out certain foods, taking supplements, and making lifestyle changes may significantly improve symptoms and quality of life.

Plus, these changes may help reduce inflammation, slow or prevent thyroid damage caused by elevated thyroid antibodies, and manage body weight, blood sugar, and cholesterol levels.

SUMMARY

Diet and lifestyle changes may significantly decrease antibody levels, improve thyroid function, and reduce symptoms caused by Hashimoto's disease.

Evidence-based dietary tips

Here are some evidence-based dietary tips to help treat Hashimoto's disease.

Gluten- and grain-free diets

Many studies indicate that those with Hashimoto's are more likely to have celiac disease than the general population. As such, experts recommend that everyone diagnosed with Hashimoto's be screened for celiac disease.

What's more, some evidence suggests that gluten- and grain-free diets may benefit people with Hashimoto's disease.

In a 6-month study in 34 women with Hashimoto's disease, a gluten-free diet reduced thyroid antibody levels while improving thyroid function and vitamin D levels, compared with a control group.

Many other studies note that people with Hashimoto's disease — or autoimmune diseases in general — likely benefit from a gluten-free diet even if they don't have celiac disease.

When following a gluten-free diet, you must avoid all wheat, barley, and rye products. For example, most pastas, breads, and soy sauces contain gluten — though gluten-free alternatives exist.

A grain-free diet is more restrictive than a gluten-free diet, as it bans all grains. Although this dietary change may also offer benefits, research supporting it is limited.

The Autoimmune Protocol Diet

The Autoimmune Protocol (AIP) Diet is designed for people with autoimmune diseases. It removes potentially harmful foods like grains, dairy, nightshades, added sugar, coffee, legumes, eggs, alcohol, nuts, seeds, refined sugars, oils, and food additives.

In a 10-week study in 16 women with Hashimoto's disease, the AIP Diet led to significant improvements in quality of life scores and significantly decreased levels of the inflammatory marker C-reactive protein (CRP).

Although these results are promising, larger longer duration studies are needed.

Keep in mind that the AIP Diet is a phased elimination diet and should be prescribed and monitored by an experienced healthcare provider.

Consider avoiding dairy

Lactose intolerance is very common among people with Hashimoto's disease.

In a study in 83 women with Hashimotos' disease, 75.9% were diagnosed with lactose intolerance.

If you suspect lactose intolerance, cutting out dairy may aid digestive issues, as well as thyroid function and medication absorption. Keep in mind that this strategy may not work for everyone, as some people with Hashimoto's tolerate dairy perfectly well.

Focus on anti-inflammatory foods

Inflammation may be a driving force behind Hashimoto's disease. As such, an anti-inflammatory diet rich in fruits and vegetables may significantly improve symptoms.

A study in 218 women with Hashimoto's disease found that markers of oxidative stress — a condition that causes chronic inflammation — were lower in those who ate fruits and vegetables more frequently.

Vegetables, fruits, spices, and fatty fish are just some examples of foods with powerful anti-inflammatory properties.

Nutrient-dense, whole foods diets

Following a diet low in added sugar and highly processed foods but rich in whole, nutrient-dense foods may help improve your health, manage your weight, and reduce Hashimoto's-related symptoms.

Whenever possible, prepare your meals at home using nutritious foods like vegetables, fruits, proteins, healthy fats, and fiber-rich carbs.

These foods offer powerful antioxidant and anti-inflammatory benefits.

Other diet tips

Some research indicates that certain low carb diets may help reduce body weight and thyroid antibodies in people with Hashimoto's disease.

These particular diets provide 12–15% of daily calories from carbs and restrict goitrogenic foods. Goitrogens are substances found in cruciferous vegetables and soy products that may interfere with thyroid hormone production.

Yet, cruciferous vegetables are highly nutritious, and cooking them diminishes their goitrogenic activity. Thus, it's unlikely that they interfere with thyroid function unless eaten in extremely large amounts.

Some evidence suggests that soy harms thyroid function as well, so many people with Hashimoto's choose to avoid soy products. Nonetheless, more research is needed.

SUMMARY

Going gluten-free, avoiding dairy, and following a nutrient-dense, anti-inflammatory diet are just a few tips that may improve symptoms of Hashimoto's disease.

Helpful supplements for Hashimoto's

Several supplements may help lower inflammation and thyroid antibodies in people with Hashimoto's disease. Plus, those with this condition are more likely to be deficient in certain nutrients, so supplementing may be necessary.

Beneficial supplements include:

• Selenium. Studies show that taking 200 mcg of selenium per day may help reduce antithyroid peroxidase (TPO) antibodies and improve well-being in people with Hashimoto's disease.

- Zinc. Zinc is essential for thyroid function. Research suggests that when used alone or alongside selenium, taking 30 mg of this mineral per day may improve thyroid function in people with hypothyroidism.

- Curcumin. Animal and human studies have shown that this powerful anti-inflammatory and antioxidant compound may protect the thyroid. Plus, it may help treat autoimmune diseases in general.

- Vitamin D. People with Hashimoto's disease have been shown to have significantly lower levels of this vitamin than the general population. What's more, studies link low vitamin D levels with Hashimoto's disease severity.

- B complex vitamins. People with Hashimoto's disease likewise tend to be low in vitamin B12. Taking a high quality B complex vitamin boosts levels of B12 and other important B vitamins (24).

- Magnesium. Low levels of this mineral are associated with an increased risk of Hashimoto's disease and higher thyroid antibodies. Plus, correcting magnesium deficiencies may improve symptoms in people with thyroid disease.

- Iron. People with Hashimoto's disease are more likely to develop anemia. Iron supplements may be needed to correct a deficiency.

Other supplements like fish oil, alpha-lipoic acid, and N-acetyl cysteine may also help people with Hashimoto's disease.

Note that supplementing with high doses of iodine in the absence of an iodine deficiency may lead to adverse effects in those with Hashimoto's. You shouldn't take high dose iodine supplements unless your healthcare provider has directed you to do so.

SUMMARY

Many vitamin and mineral supplements, including zinc, vitamin D, and magnesium, may benefit those with Hashimoto's disease.

Foods to eat

If you have Hashimoto's disease, a nutrient-dense diet may help reduce the severity of your symptoms and improve your overall health. Focus on the following foods:

- Fruits: berries, pears, apples, peaches, citrus fruits, pineapple, bananas, etc.

- Non-starchy vegetables: zucchini, artichokes, tomatoes, asparagus, carrots, peppers, broccoli, arugula, mushrooms, etc.

- Starchy vegetables: sweet potatoes, potatoes, peas, acorn and butternut squash, etc.

- Healthy fats: avocados, avocado oil, coconut oil, olive oil, unsweetened coconut flakes, full fat yogurt, coconut yogurt, etc.

- Animal protein: salmon, eggs, cod, turkey, shrimp, chicken, etc.

- Gluten-free grains: brown rice, rolled oats, quinoa, brown rice pasta, etc.

- Seeds, nuts, and nut butters: cashews, almonds, macadamia nuts, sunflower seeds, pumpkin seeds, natural peanut butter, almond butter, etc.

- Beans and lentils: chickpeas, black beans, lentils, etc.

- Dairy and nondairy substitutes (fortified with calcium and/or vitamin D): coconut milk, coconut yogurt, almond milk, cashew milk, full fat unsweetened yogurt, goat cheese, etc.

- Spices, herbs, and condiments: turmeric, basil, rosemary, paprika, saffron, black pepper, salsa, tahini, honey, lemon juice, apple cider vinegar, etc.

- Beverages: water, unsweetened tea, sparkling water, etc.

Keep in mind that some people with Hashimoto's disease avoid a few of the foods mentioned above, such as grains and dairy. It's important to experiment with your diet to find out what foods work best for you.

SUMMARY

Whole, nutrient-dense foods should make up the majority of any healthy diet and may be especially helpful if you have Hashimoto's disease.

Foods to avoid

Eliminating or restricting the following foods may help reduce Hashimoto's symptoms and improve your overall health:

• Added sugars and sweets: soda, energy drinks, cakes, ice cream, pastries, cookies, candy, sugary cereals, table sugar, etc.

• Fast food and fried foods: french fries, hot dogs, fried chicken, etc.

• Refined grains: white pasta, white bread, white flour tortillas, bagels, etc.

• Highly processed foods and meats: frozen dinners, margarine, microwave dinners, bacon, sausage, etc.

• Gluten-containing grains and foods: wheat, barley, rye, crackers, bread, etc.

Some healthcare providers suggest that people with Hashimoto's disease avoid soy and dairy as well — and sometimes even nightshades and all grains.

However, although these recommendations may help many individuals, it's important to experiment with your diet to find the best method for you.

Working with a dietitian who specializes in autoimmune diseases like Hashimoto's disease can help you narrow down potentially problematic foods and set up an eating pattern that'll help you feel your best.

SUMMARY

Steering clear of added sugar, highly processed foods, and gluten-containing grains may help reduce Hashimoto's symptoms and improve your overall health.

Other lifestyle modifications to try

Getting plenty of sleep, reducing stress, and practicing self-care are extremely important for those with Hashimoto's disease.

In fact, research shows that engaging in stress reduction practices helps reduce depression and anxiety, improve overall quality of life, and lower thyroid antibodies in women with Hashimoto's disease.

Letting your body rest when you're feeling fatigued is important as well.

Additionally, you should take thyroid medication on an empty stomach at least 30–60 minutes before breakfast or at least 3–4 hours after dinner for maximum absorption.

Even coffee and dietary supplements interfere with thyroid medication absorption, so it's best to consume nothing but water for at least 30 minutes after taking your medicine.

Your healthcare provider can answer any questions about how to ensure maximum absorption.

Keep in mind that when you're first starting medication, it may take a few weeks or longer to start feeling better. If your symptoms aren't improving, speak to your healthcare provider about other options.

As Hashimoto's symptoms may significantly affect your quality of life and mental health, be sure to find a healthcare team that you trust. This may take some time, but it's essential to getting the right treatment.

SUMMARY

Reducing stress, getting plenty of rest, and practicing self-care are essential for those with Hashimoto's disease. Finding a healthcare provider whom you trust is also key.

Diagnosis and symptoms

It's thought that Hashimoto's disease develops from an immune defect coupled with environmental factors, though these factors aren't fully understood.

Diagnosis depends on symptoms and laboratory results.

Lab results indicating Hashimoto's disease include elevated thyroid-stimulating hormone (TSH), low levels of free thyroxine (FT4), and increased anti-thyroid peroxidase (anti-TPO) antibodies.

Some people with Hashimoto's disease also have elevated TSH receptor-blocking antibodies (TBII) and antithyroglobulin (anti-Tg) antibodies. These antibodies attack the thyroid gland (1Trusted Source).

The disease's destruction of the thyroid is intermittent. During its early stages, people may present with symptoms and lab results that indicate hyperthyroidism — or even have normal lab values.

As such, Hashimoto's disease is often difficult to detect, and individuals may go for months without the proper diagnosis. Up to one-third of people treated for hypothyroidism don't receive adequate or proper treatment.

Hashimoto's disease affects both women and men, but women are 5–10 times more likely to be diagnosed. Your risk increases with age, and most women are diagnosed between the ages of 30 and 50.

This condition is usually treated with synthetic or natural thyroid hormones. Synthetic ones include levothyroxine (Synthroid) and liothyronine (Cytomel), while natural ones include Armour Thyroid and Naturethroid.

Symptoms

Because Hashimoto's disease affects nearly every organ system in your body, it's associated with a variety of symptoms. These include (1Trusted Source, 51Trusted Source):

- weight gain

- extreme fatigue

- poor concentration

- thinning, coarse hair

- dry skin

- slow or irregular heart rate

- decreased muscle strength

- shortness of breath

- decreased exercise tolerance

- cold intolerance

- elevated blood pressure

- brittle nails

- constipation

- neck pain or thyroid tenderness

- depression and anxiety

- menstrual irregularities

- insomnia

- voice changes

Untreated or improperly treated Hashimoto's disease may lead to serious side effects, such as an increased risk of heart disease, cognitive disorders, and even death.

SUMMARY

Hashimoto's symptoms vary widely and include weight gain, fatigue, cold intolerance, and constipation. The disease is diagnosed based on symptoms and lab results.

The bottom line

Hashimoto's disease is a common autoimmune condition that affects the thyroid. It causes numerous symptoms that may persist even if you take thyroid medication.

Research shows that dietary and lifestyle changes can significantly improve your symptoms and boost your overall health. However, every person with Hashimoto's disease is different, so it's fundamental to find a dietary pattern that suits your needs.

A dietitian or other healthcare provider who specializes in autoimmune diseases may be able to help you find an eating pattern that works for

you.

9 798857 740934